The exhiLarate 10-steps to a Healthier - and Happier - You

I0411423

Lara Foldvari

Legal stuff you probably won't read:

I am not a medical doctor. I am also not a registered dietician, or a physical therapist. For anything beyond the scope of this book, please refer to the proper professional. Any advice given is to be taken on the knowledge that it is from a certified personal trainer and lifestyle & weight management specialist with personal experience.

YoLarates™ is trademarked. Don't use the name. It's mine.

If you want to copy anything from this book, go ahead. Just give me credit, 'kay?

Acknowledgements

Sometimes people will say or do something major that will affect your life and how you live it; sometimes it's seemingly minor, but still packs a punch. These folks have molded who I am today in regards to how I look at food and exercise:

My Mom and Dad sent me off to my first ballet lesson at the Rene Jennings School of Dance when I was just four years old. For the next dozen years they spent thousands of dollars and countless hours carting me to classes at the Boston Ballet, and then the Connecticut Ballet schools. I was never the best in my class, but Mom and Dad knew I loved it, and they always encouraged me. My love of dance is thanks to them. Thank you, Mom and Dad!!

Mom and Dad also had me eating right, right from the start. Whatever they were having for dinner, that's what my sister and I had. There was no separate meal of chicken nuggets and tater tots for us. If they were having Weiner Schnitzel, rice pilaf and Brussels sprouts, that's what we had, too. We regularly ate at Chinese restaurants, but a trip to McDonald's was a very rare treat. And we didn't know what cola was until I was four years old and we were in Hungary. My *nagymama* had stocked her tiny 'fridge with Pepsi cola because she thought all American kids drank it. When we returned home, I asked my parents if they had Pepsi in America and they lied (!) and said "no." To this day, McDonald's is a once or twice a year event, as is cola.

I have a few men in my life who gave me jolts. The first was my soulmate, Bruce Owen. When I was a tender 14 years old, he told me that my breasts would be hanging to my knees by the time I was 40. He believes that this wildly inappropriate comment is why I have preserved myself so well. I'll give him credit for this if he wants it because I love him.

His friend, Bondo, also shocked me into doing something about my figure when he basically told me I was fat and needed his wife's expertise.

Speaking of Bondo's wife... thank you, Annalisa, for your support when I was chubby, for providing a place for me to teach, and for your friendship! *Grazie*!

Thank you to my ballet instructors at the Connecticut Ballet, especially Robin Welch and Robert Vickery, who treated all of their dancers and students with respect; and to Allyson Barker who made me cry, but pushed me to do my best.

My students and my clients; what can I say? You show up every week and allow me to see how far YOU have come in your own health and fitness journeys. Being a positive influence in others' lives is why I do what I do, so THANK YOU for letting me do that for you!

And to my proofreaders: thank you for making what I had to say more clear so that I can help even one more person to become healthy and fit!

Table of Contents

The exhiLarate 10-steps to a Healthier (and happier!) You

Notice that this is not the "1-step to a skinny you" program. While getting healthy means, for many of us, to lose weight, it's more than that. There are plenty of skinny fat people out there who are thin because they starve themselves and live on cigarettes and coffee. But are they healthy? Or happy? If a byproduct of this program is weight loss, consider it a bonus; it is not the goal.

This is the beginning of your new healthier and happier life. Ten steps. I used to offer this as a 10-week program, but I'd prefer to give you all of the tools you need up front, and let YOU decide how you are going to do this. However, after a few years of fine-tuning the program, I can tell you that this has been the most logical and effective path.

Here are the steps. While I give you the steps, you are the one who has to follow them. But as you will read in my background, I did these myself.

1. Why do you want to get healthy? What are some of your goals?

2. Get yourself a support system!

3. Goals and organization!

4. Let's go to the grocery store

5. Re-make your recipes

6. Get moving!

7. De-stress and focus on YOU

8. Don't be afraid of restaurants

9. ... or holidays

10. How are you going to stay on track?

Let me introduce myself.

"Hi! I'm Lara, and I'm just like you." If you've read my cookbook, *Just a Good Cook...*, you might recognize these words. In that book, I let you know that I was not a professional cook; just an average homemaker (just like you). Now I am telling you that I am not an athlete; I am not a fitness model; I am an average middle-age homemaker. However, I am a healthy one. Not all of us can say that, and I am here to help change that for you.

Unlike in my cookbook, where I tell you I have no professional chef training, I do have some national certifications in health and wellness. I am ACE, AFAA, NESTA & NASM certified as a personal trainer, group fitness instructor, lifestyle and weight management specialist, and fitness nutrition specialist. Besides these "official" qualifications, I also have practical experience in helping friends and clients to lose weight, eat better, start (and continue) exercising, and, bottom-line, get healthier.

I am also my own best testimonial.

As a (very) young girl, my parents started me in ballet classes because my legs were too skinny. Classmates referred to me as "small fry" and "shrimp," and I was always the last person picked for a team in phys ed.

I was able to eat whatever I wanted because I was dancing every day. Until I broke my toe when I was 14. That's when the bacon and French fries and Cokes started to take effect. I was no longer skinny, and I went off to college at a healthy 120 pounds on my 5'4" frame.

By Christmas break I was 130. My boyfriend called me "thunder thighs."

I dropped out of college and married a drug addict. Stress and cigarettes brought my weight down to an all-time adult-Lara low of 105 pounds.

I got divorced and gained 20 much-needed pounds. Married a second time and gained another 20. It took another divorce to lose those 20.

Are you doing the math? I got up to 125, then 145, then came back down to 125.

What an unhealthy roller-coaster! Not only was my weight fluctuating, so were my cholesterol counts. I had also been diagnosed with fibromyalgia in my late 20's, and as I gained weight, I gained pain, too.

So why did I allow myself, at 39 years old, to pack on not 20 pounds, but 35 pounds?!? That's just when our metabolism is really starting to slow down.

By my 40th birthday, a friend suggested that I go to his wife for personal training because he used to be able to grab my ass with one hand, and now he needed two. Ouch!

I decided to do it on my own. I ditched the mixed drinks for wine spritzers. I started eating the reduced-fat versions of full-fat foods. I got on the treadmill, and then started working out to my dozens of exercise DVDs. It took a good six months, but by the summer, I was back down to 125 pounds.

That was five years ago. My weight fluctuates a few pounds above and below that, but for the most part, I've maintained this.

I eat. I drink. I *don't* kill myself working out.

People see me at parties, eating and drinking – a lot- and ask me how I do it. They think I must starve myself the rest of the time to be able to eat like that. Or they think that I live at the gym. Neither is the case.

However, it IS a balancing act. Not 50/50, but 80/20.

80 percent of the time, I eat really well. This makes up for the 20 percent that consists of wine, chocolate, pizza, and other treats.

Also, 80% of keeping our weight in check is diet. Only 20% is exercise.

But you DO need to exercise! I happen to have hypothyroidism (an underactive thyroid gland), which means that my metabolism needs an extra boost. We should all work on making our metabolism rev as much as possible. Cardio and weight training combined is the magic.

So you see, I am a real person. Just like you.

I do real exercise. No Olympic weight training or boot camps (because I'm not heading to the Olympics or the military). Exercise, for the majority of us, should be safe and effective (and fun!).

I eat real food. No shakes as meal replacements. No fat-free, low-carb, leaving-out-entire-food-groups. Real FOOD.

Be patient. You didn't become overweight or unhealthy overnight, and you certainly aren't going to reverse things immediately, either. You saw my track record. It took 20 years of my weight fluctuating wildly before I got myself under control.

I don't want you to have to spend as much time as I did, wading through information that often contradicts the last "fact" you learned. There's no need (unless you desire) to spend the time and money that I did taking courses and earning certifications.

Follow the steps and you will succeed!

I have a real life. A really healthy and happy one. You can, too.

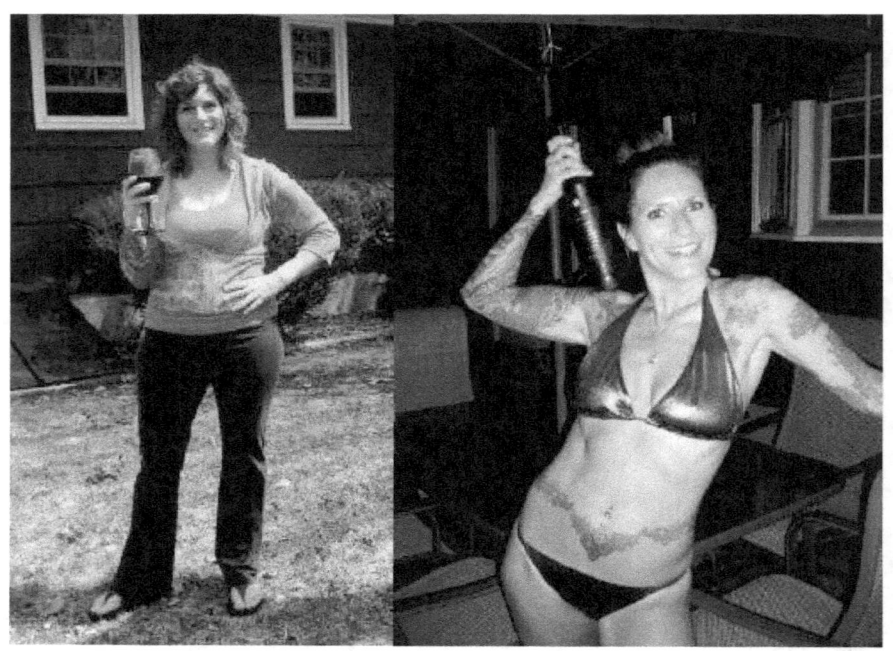

Lara at 160+ pounds and at approximately 125 pounds

Step One

So, tell me, what brought you here? Losing weight is a great goal, but I want you to think about gaining health instead of losing weight.

Why do you want to get healthy? How are you going to measure your health goals? Lower cholesterol? Lower BMI? Lower number on the scale?

Make sure these goals are specific! "I will have my cholesterol under 200." "I will lose 15 pounds by May 15th."

I'm asking questions that you will have to answer for yourself.

What do you like to eat? What don't you like to eat? Who cares? You do! If you are trying to eat healthy, don't put yourself on a cabbage diet if you hate cabbage. I know carboholics who are trying to succeed with a Paleo (very-low-carb) diet. I know carnivores who are attempting to be healthy by going Vegan (no animal products at all). You will have no LONG TERM success if you try to eat against your dietary grain (pardon the low-carb pun). And for the short term while you might be making progress with this diet, you likely would be miserable.

What good is being healthy if you aren't happy?

So do me a favor, please, and do not cut entire food groups out of your diet. OK? (Caveat- food allergies. Please DO cut out scallops if you are allergic to shellfish!)

Since exercise is 20% of what you need to do, what has your experience been with exercise? Here's a personal story to give you an idea of what I'm asking: I was terrified to learn how to ride a bicycle. I finally did, but I never felt truly comfortable on one. When I was 21, I almost passed out after riding a stationary bicycle at the gym. At 31, I wiped out while riding my bike with my boyfriend, and then tearfully broke up with him. At 41 I took a spin class and couldn't walk the next day. Clearly, two-wheeled exercise is not for me.

But ballet, ah, that's a different story. I put on ballet slippers at age four and haven't looked back. Gyms scare the heck out of me, and I won't get much return on any investment I put into going to one. Because I won't go. But I can walk into any dance studio and feel at home.

So think back on YOUR experiences. Even if it's a simple as neighborhood kickball that you loved, or walking your dog. When we get moving in Step Six, you're going to want to know how you like to move.

Finally, I insist that you join MyFitnessPal (www.myfitnesspal.com). You must write down everything you eat. You must track your exercise. Get yourself a fitbit (www.fitbit.com). I use both of these, and if you want to see what I eat and do for exercise, join these and become friends with me on the sites. I love to share with you!

In general, most of us should be aiming for something like this as far as macronutrient numbers go:

Total calories: 1650

Fat: 50 g

Protein: 100g

Carbs: 200 g

Fiber: 20 g

These are numbers to be looking for while you are tracking your food intake. Everyone is different, so this is just a guideline.*

Think these things over:

- Eat your breakfast!

- Eat 5-6 small meals instead of three large ones

- Drink water! About half as many ounces of your weight in pounds. For example, if you are 120 pounds, drink 60 ounces of water a day, more if you are exercising heavily or it is hot outside

- Write it down! What you eat, how you move, and how you feel

- Treat yourself! Don't think of them as "cheats," think of them as "treats."

- Do both cardio and weight training

- Be kind to yourself

Fill out this questionnaire. When I meet with clients in person, we go over this together. If you answer "yes" to any of the "History" questions, I urge you to have a physical, or at least see a physician, before embarking on any exercise program.

*For individualized micro- and macronutrient needs, please consult a Registered Dietician

HEALTH & MEDICAL QUESTIONNAIRE

Name: _____

Date of birth: _____

Date: _____

Address:_____

Street

City   State   Zip

Phone (Cell): _____ (Work): _____

Email address: _____

In case of emergency, whom may we contact?

Name: _____

Relationship: _____

Phone (Cell):_____

(Home):_____

Personal physician

Name: _____

Phone: _____

Fax: _____

Present/Past History

Have you had or do you presently have any of the following? (Check if yes.)

_____ Rheumatic fever

_____ Recent operation

_____ Edema (swelling of ankles)

_____ High blood pressure

_____ Low blood pressure

_____ Injury to back or knees

_____ Seizures

_____ Lung disease

_____ Heart attack or known heart disease

_____ Fainting or dizziness

_____ Diabetes

_____ High Cholesterol

_____ Orthopnea (the need to sit up to breathe comfortably) or paroxysmal (sudden, unexpected attack) or nocturnal dyspnea (shortness of breath at night)

_____ Shortness of breath at rest or with mild exertion

_____ Chest pains

_____ Palpitations or tachycardia (unusually strong or rapid beat)

_____ Intermittent claudication (calf cramping)

_____ Pain, discomfort in the chest, neck, jaw, arms, or other areas

_____ Known heart murmur

_____ Unusual fatigue or shortness of breath with usual activities

_____ Temporary loss of visual acuity or speech, or short-term numbness or weakness in one side, arm, or leg of your body

_____ Cancer

_____ Other (please describe):

_____

Family History

Have any of your first-degree relatives (parent, sibling, or child) experienced the following conditions? (Check if yes.) In addition, please identify at what age the condition occurred.

_____ Heart attack

_____ Heart operation (Bypass surgery, Angioplasty, Coronary Stent placement)

_____ Congenital heart disease

_____ High blood pressure

_____ High cholesterol

_____ Diabetes

_____ Other major illness:

_____

Explain checked items :

_____
_____
_____
_____
_____

Activity History

1. How were you referred to this program? (Please be specific.)
   _____

2. Why are you enrolling in this program? (Please be specific.)
   _____

3. Have you ever worked with a personal trainer before?
   Yes ___ No ___

4. Date of your last physical examination performed by a physician: _____

5. Do you participate in a regular exercise program at this time?
   Yes _____ No _____ If yes, briefly describe:
   _____
   _____
   _____

5. Can you currently walk 4 miles briskly without fatigue?
   Yes ___ No _____

6. Have you ever performed resistance training exercises in the past?
   Yes _____ No _____

7. Do you have injuries (bone or muscle disabilities) that may interfere with exercising? Yes _____ No _____ If yes, briefly describe:
   _____

8. Do you smoke? Yes _____ No _____ If yes, how much per day and what was your age when you started? Amount per day _____ Age _____

9. What is your body weight now? _____ What was it one year ago? _____
   At age 21? _____

10. How tall are you? ___

11. Do you follow or have you recently followed any specific dietary intake plan and, in general, how do you feel about your nutritional habits?

_____

_____

_____

_____

12. List the medications you are presently taking (including street drugs.

_____

_____

_____

_____

13. List in order your personal health and fitness objectives.
    a. _____
    b. _____
    c. _____
    d. _____

Step Two

I want to know what obstacles you might've had in the past and have you enlisted a support system?

Obstacles might include not having enough time or money (set the alarm 30 minutes before you normally do and take a walk or do an exercise DVD); or having a crazy travel schedule for work (bring exercise DVDs on the road with you and pack healthy foods); or having too many social obligations (see Steps Eight and Nine) ; or an unhealthy group of friends and family (see below).

Your husband, kids, coworkers, friends, and more, are good support systems. You know what else is? A group fitness class! I'm not just saying this to get more people into my YoLarates™ and Zumba® classes. Your fellow classmates probably have similar goals as you do. Instead of competing with each other, I've found that people who join in group fitness classes support and encourage one another. Try to hit one up at least once a week.

Cooking classes can also be a great way to meet other like-minded people. Just make sure that they are HEALTHY cooking classes!

You are already signed up on MyFitnessPal (right??), and you're recording everything you are eating (right??), but did you also know that you can use the site for support? Become friends on the site with your Facebook friends. Click on the "Community" tab and find all kinds of support.

Even if you don't have "live" people in your life who are supporting your efforts, you can definitely find cyber-support!

I also want to suggest some books that you might want to check out/purchase, some free websites to go to, and apps to download right now. For books, I highly recommend *Frumpy to Fabulous* by Josette Puig. She gives you a change a week, and it's amazing what those simple changes can do. A similar book, by the clean-eating queen Tosca Reno, is *Just the Rules!* It includes 51 rules, so you can parallel this with Josette's book.

There are three pocket guides which I either carry with me or keep close, that I think you should, too. Lisa Lillien's *Hungry Girl Supermarket Survival Aisle By Aisle, HG-Style* is a must for the grocery shopping that we will be doing in Week Four.

Rocco DiSpirito's *Now Eat This! 100 Quick Calorie Cuts* is an often-consulted guide for me, especially when I am heading to a restaurant (as we will in Week Eight).

Finally, The Calorie King®'s *Fat & Carbohydrate Counter*. This guide is updated yearly, so find the most recent one and carry it with you!

For good recipes that are make-overs of comfort food, I like Rocco DiSpirito's *Now Eat This*. The mac and cheese is awesome! Also, my cookbook, *Just a Good Cook...* has lots of cleaned-up recipes.

All can be found on amazon.com.

As for websites, check out Lisa Lillien, the Hungry Girl: http://www.hungry-girl.com/ Her newsletter is great! LOTS of tips and tricks for eating. There are some recipes that use not-so-clean ingredients, but if you are just starting out, just learning how to make adjustments in what you eat can be very helpful.

Bookmark www.CalorieKing.com to access the most updated Counter.

Recipes can be found at www.Sparkpeople.com, which is a terrific site.

The Calorie King® and Sparkpeople® both have apps that you really should download onto your smartphone. Other apps are Fooducate, which you can use at the grocery store, and ChallengeLoop, to find fitness challenges that you might want to join (great support, hint hint).

Whatever you do, be your own cheerleader, and don't let anyone try to discourage you from your goals!

Step Three

You've set your goals, right? Without goals you can't know what you are aiming for. And without a plan, you won't be able to achieve your goals. I finally figured this out last year, and WOW, what a difference it has made in all aspects of my life!

I learned about setting goals through Chalene Johnson, and she learned through Brian Tracy, so I recommend going to them for the best advice and outlines on how to set, and achieve, goals.

They also help with organization, and I've picked up tips from them, but you can always search out your own experts. If you don't feel comfortable with, or can't relate to a certain expert, then find another one. There are plenty out there!

So, you need to organize your goals, and you need to be organized in general. Being organized takes away so much stress.

What follows is how I have set goals and how I organize my life. I really cannot emphasize enough how important it is to have goals and to be organized!

My first organizational piece is my calendar. Just a good ol' fashioned wall calendar. It's hanging in my kitchen (the hub of my home) and is referred to many times a day.

This is not the place to put every single thing that you do every single day. For that you will use a day planner or a calendar app on your smartphone. The wall calendar is for deviations from your normal schedule, appointments, and special events.

I have my current ever-changing work schedule under the wall calendar. If you work different shifts, this helps to keep you, and your family members, in sync with where you will be and when.

As for those day planners, they can be on your smartphone or on paper. I keep both, mostly because I am a sucker for office products and journals. But whatever you feel that you will use, chose that, and USE it. Keep it current and refer to it often.

Other ways to stay organized include using labeled file folders for projects, jobs, events, and more. I currently have folders for every step in this program, one for each volunteer group that I work with, recipes that I want to try, and my upcoming vacation.

I keep these current folders in the kitchen, which is where I tend to do most of my work. Less-frequently used folders, such as those for yearly events, are kept in an open file box in my less-used office.

Do what works for YOU. Color-coding, file boxes, notebooks, and even neat piles might work better for you. Find your soulmate organizational system and stick to it!

Step Four

Hopefully you will be doing the bulk of your eating at home. Not only is this more economical, but you have way more control over what you eat.

But what to buy? And where?

If you have a Trader Joe's or a Whole Foods near you, start there. (They are sometimes, but not always, pricier than the grocery store, but your health is worth it, and you'll likely save more in lower medical bills in the long run.) You have a much better chance of finding clean food. Notice I didn't say "low calorie" or "low fat" or "low carb" or any other restrictive description. Food is your friend and we've spent far too many years fearing it or hating it.

Farms and small local health food stores are also terrific for organic and special regional foods.

Most of us, most of the time, will be heading to the big box grocery store. And that's fine, especially now-a-days since their natural foods sections tend to be expanding. Yay!

Some tips: don't shop if you are hungry, and only get what is on your shopping list! If you head into the grocery store famished, you'll be more likely to walk out with Oreos. Don't do it! You're doing this for yourself and for your family, and if it isn't in the house, you (and your family members) won't be able to eat it.

Feel free to copy my shopping list. These are items that I regularly purchase and keep on hand at home.

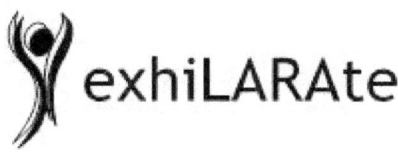

The exhiLarate 10-steps to health grocery shopping list

Fruits

Avocados

Apples

Bananas

Berries (blueberries, raspberries, strawberries, blackberries)

Grapefruit

Lemons

Limes

Oranges

Pears

Tomatoes

Frozen fruits & vegetable mixes

Veggies

Garlic

Cucumber

Onions

Lettuce (Romaine, Boston, Iceberg)

Spinach

Kales

Asparagus

Broccoli

Celery

Potatoes

Sweet Potatoes

Squash (Summer, Zucchini, Spaghetti, Acorn)

Mushrooms

Green Beans

Beets

Bell peppers (red, green, yellow, orange)

Herbs (basil, cilantro, parsley, mint, chives, rosemary)

Meats

Boneless, skinless chicken breasts

Pork chops

Steaks (Porterhouse, sirloin, tenderloin, flank)

Lean ground beef (at least 90% lean)

Lean ground turkey meat

Turkey or chicken kielbasa

Other turkey or chicken sausages

White fish (tilapia, halibut, cod, red snapper)

Bacon, center cut

Dairy

Skim milk

Almond milk

Coconut milk

Eggs

Fat-free Greek yogurt

Reduced fat shredded cheeses (Cheddar, Mexican blend, Italian blend, Mozzarella)

Reduced fat block cheeses (made with 2% milk or 50% or 75% fat-free)

Low-fat sour cream

Low-fat cream cheese

Low-fat cottage cheese

Farmer's cheese

Butter, unsalted

Slow-churned ice cream

Frozen Greek yogurt

Grains

White whole wheat flour

Brown rice (short, long, Basmati, Jasmine)

Quinoa

Couscous

Barley

Bulgur

Millet

Amaranth

Buckwheat

High-fiber pasta

Sprouted grain breads

Whole grain, low-carb tortilla wraps

Rolled oats

Kasha Go Lean cereals

Weetabix cereal

Cream of Wheat (farina)

Other high fiber, low-fat, low-sugar cereals

Herbs & Spices

Hungarian sweet paprika

Cumin

Madras curry powder

Crushed red pepper

Spike seasoning

Fines Herbes

Herbs de Provence

Nutmeg

Cinnamon

Vanilla extract

Fats (oils & nuts)

Almonds, walnuts, pecans, cashews, peanuts

All-natural nut butters

Powdered peanut butter

Extra virgin olive oil

Coconut oil

Shredded coconut

Canned goods

Stock & broth

Beans! (black, pinto, cannellini, chick peas, lentils, kidney)

Crushed or chopped tomatoes

Tomato paste

Rotel (tomatoes & green chilies)

Olives

White tuna in water

Clams & clam juice

Artichoke hearts

Low-sodium soups

And the rest

Mustards

Salsa

Honey

Maple syrup

Agave nectar

Stevia

Vinegar (apple, wine, rice, balsamic)

Bragg's Liquid Aminos

Low-sodium soy sauce

Ponzu sauce

Coconut water

Coconut milk

Dark chocolate

Step Five

Now that you have all that clean, healthy food, you have to cook it! There are TONS of cookbooks and websites and apps with recipes that are healthy AND delicious (these need not be mutually exclusive!). Here are my favorites:

Books:

Any of Rocco DiSpirito's *Now Eat This!* cookbooks

Any of Tosca Reno's *Eat-Clean Diet* cookbooks

Any of Lisa Lillien's *Hungry Girl* cookbooks

App:

SparkRecipes

Once you get the hang of it, you'll be making the swaps yourself and not even thinking about it. Here are my Quick tips:

- Water, Water, Water

- Eat slower

- Lean proteins, such as fish, chicken, pork and lean cuts of beef

    - Beans and tofu as vegetarian options

- Watch your portions

- Use oatmeal instead of bread crumbs

- Wine for flavor instead of fat

- Veggies to bulk up recipes

- Low-fat dairy

- Bake instead of frying

- Snack on celery

- Use onions and garlic and herbs and spices

- Salt adds flavor without adding fat (just don't use too much)

- Egg whites or a combo of whites with one yolk

- Greek yogurt in place of sour cream (or combine the two)

- Evaporated milk instead of cream (awesome for making white sauces)

- Spray your oil instead of pouring it

- Pungent cheeses go a long way, so you can use less (parmesan, blue)

- Use center cut bacon

- Salsa on everything (pasta, eggs, baked potatoes)

- Stevia instead of sugar or artificial sweeteners

- Whole grain pasta. Slightly OVER-cook it. (I know! NOT al dente! Trust me!)

- In a pinch for dinner? Make breakfast. Eggs, Canadian bacon, rye toast and an orange.

Step Six

You need to get moving! Yes, what you eat is 80% of it, but 20% is exercise, and you are in this 100 percent, right? Right!

Think back to your past exercise experience. What was successful for you in the past? Pick that up again!

No exercise history? You have SO many options! Here's how I suggest you get started. Take a walk. Throw on a pair of sneakers and hit the pavement. Unless you are bound to a wheelchair, you can walk. It might not be as far or for as long a time as you'd like, but if you are mobile, you can take a walk.

I'm a huge fan of group fitness classes because of the moral support that can be found in them, and also because they tend to be fun. You're probably not going to stick with an exercise program if it isn't fun. Get a one-week pass to a local fitness center and start taking classes. Any class that remotely speaks to you, take it!

Your local Parks & Rec and Adult Education programs probably offer a variety of classes that you can check out without joining a gym. Sign up for one. Or two.

If you are shy, or intimidated by large gyms, or feel like you'd embarrass yourself in a class, consider hiring a personal trainer. Yes, this can be costly, but you can start with a couple sessions and see how it goes from there. You don't have to marry him or her. (As a personal trainer, I can tell you that it's not my goal to keep you as a client forever. I want to give you the tools to be able to work out on your own.) One bonus of meeting with a personal trainer is that you will learn how to do exercises properly, making your workouts safer and more effective. (Make sure your trainer has a *current* certification from ACSM, NASM, ACE, AFAA, or another national certification, and has a *current* CPR/AED certification, and is insured.)

There are also thousands of exercise DVDs that you can purchase or even rent from the library. I love to hate Jillian Michaels. While I don't agree with making people work out so hard that they puke, she *is* motivating. Any of the Beachbody® programs are excellent. P90X® is popular for a reason- it works. Personally, I love Brazil Butt Lift® and ChaLEAN Extreme®, but you have to find what YOU love. Borrow a friend's set of DVDs so you can to try out the program.

Then, there's YouTube. Type in a workout name and you'll be brought to more snippets than you need to get a taste of what the workout will be like. You can even find entire, full-length videos of some.

Finally, I don't like Sparkpeople® only for recipes, I also like their detailed selection of exercises and workouts. Here are my favorites for beginners:

Upper Body:

biceps curls (dumbbells or band)
chest press (dumbbells or band)
dumbbell flys
dumbbell lateral raises
modified pushups
triceps dips with bent knees

Lower Body:

bridges
calf raises (wall or chair)
dumbbell squats
forward lunges
lateral lunges
lying leg curls
seated leg extensions
wide leg squats with dumbbell

Core:

crunches
crunches with twist
modified plank
modified side plank
reverse crunch
swimming

For Stretching, do these:

camel
cat
child's Pose
neck Stretch
standing chest stretch
standing shoulder stretch
seated hip and glute
leaning single leg calf stretch at wall
standing modified forward bend
standing modified hamstring stretch
standing quad stretch
torso twist

Do the stretches after the exercises. Warm up for 5-10 minutes before doing the strength exercises. You can walk, run up and down stairs, jump rope, etc. Start with 1 set of 8-12 reps of each exercise.

Step Seven

Stress in unavoidable. No matter who you are, you are gonna have stress in your life. You want to learn how to have less stress (being a more organized and healthier you is gonna help with this) and how to manage the stress that you are left with.

Stress can equal a surge in cortisol which can lead to your body holding on to the weight you are trying to get rid of. Stress can raise your blood pressure, make you (and those around you) miserable, and can wear down your immune system, among other things.

Here are some ways to de-stress:

1. Drink more water

2. Drink a cup of tea (especially chamomile)

3. Breathe; deep breaths with full exhales

4. Step outside

5. Take a walk

6. Pop a piece of cheese (low-fat)

7. Indulge in a piece (or two) of dark chocolate

8. Jump or hop

9. Tense all your muscles, then relax them

10. Read a book

11. Take a nap

12. Call a friend (or mom or sister)

13. Be grateful

14. Get a massage

15. Play a board game

16. Write in a journal

17. Watch your posture

18. Chew gum

19. Make a to-do list

20. Meditate/yoga

21. Delegate tasks

22. Make time for a hobby

23. Do a forward-bend (standing or sitting)

24. Watch comedy clips (or movie)

25. Take a hot bath or shower

26. Un-plug from technology

Step Eight

I used to love eating out at restaurants. Then, when I was on a restrictive diet, I hated it. I now have a healthy relationship with restaurants. Going out for dinner is a treat. (Side bar: notice I said "treat." I abhor the term "cheat" since it's so negative. You are treating yourself, not cheating on something!) Just be prepared.

When you go out to eat:

1. Check the menu online first if you can, and try to get an idea of the healthy items you'll order
2. Drink a lot of water before, during, and after the meal
3. Start with soup- NOT cream-based
4. Just say "no" to the bread-and-butter (send the basket back)
5. Get your salad dressing on the side, then dip your fork into it first, and then your salad
6. Stay away from breaded, fried, crispy, butter, cream
7. Eat your veggies (you can ask for extra veggies instead of starchy side dish)
8. Lean protein on your plate (chicken, fish, lean beef and pork)
9. Split a dessert and then just have a bite or two

When at McDonald's:

A plain hamburger is actually better than the grilled chicken sandwich. Grilled chicken is better than nuggets.
Get a salad with dressing on the side.
Ask for kid's size or half of a small order of fries.

At Subway:

They make it simple: choose one of the low-fat sandwiches or salads (they are marked with that little American Heart Association Heart-Check symbol).

At the Chinese take-out:

Skip:

anything fried or crispy (General Tso's chicken, egg rolls, fried wontons)
Kung Pao chicken
spare ribs
fried rice

Eat:

chicken with mushrooms
steamed chicken & broccoli
clear soups
lo mein with vegetables or shrimp
moo goo gai pan (it's chicken with veggies)
moo shi
Szechuan green beans

Pizza:

if you can, get it on a whole wheat crust
ask for less cheese
load with veggies instead of meat

Step Nine

Holidays (and parties) happen. And not just Halloween, Thanksgiving, and Christmas. We have entire seasons of holidays, namely Memorial Day through Labor Day, and Halloween through New Year's Eve. It's easy to get caught up in the moment and over-indulge. Indulging here and there is good for you (remember, it's a TREAT), but when you over-do it, well, it probably starts to feel a little like cheating…

So, what to do? You can't politely refuse every invite, especially when it's something like your favorite aunt's 100th birthday celebration. You CAN have your cake and eat it too!

Social gathering how-tos:

1. Do not go hungry! Have a bowl of broth and a huge glass of water before you hit the event. You'll be less likely to immediately devour everything in sight.

2. No parking! Don't park yourself close to the buffet table. Make it difficult to refill your plate.

3. Choose a little bit of everything. Yes. Have everything that you want to have. Just have a LITTLE of it. Take one stuffed mushroom, not three of them. One cookie, not a half dozen. One SLICE of pizza, not an entire pie.

4. Choose a lot of a little. Load your plate with veggies. They'll fill you up, leaving little room for bon-bons and other nutritionally empty foods.

5. Bottoms up! Water, that is. If you are going to have wine, make it a spritzer (club soda or seltzer), ask for a skinny margarita instead of a monstrous frozen concoction, a light beer instead of regular, and a bottle of water instead of a can of soda (even the diet stuff is evil!)

6. Bring a dish. Make one (or two) of your healthy recipes and share them with your friends and family.

7. Socialize. If you were taught any manners, you know not to talk with your mouth full. So keep talking, and laughing! (Bonus, you probably won't notice that red velvet cake that's being brought out...)

8. Dance, dance, dance! You'll be so busy burning calories that you won't have time to eat, or drink, more.

9. Duck out early. Go home. No one likes a hanger-on anyway. Plus, you need your beauty sleep.

Step Ten

You now have all the basic information that you need to get healthy. But getting healthy is just the beginning. This isn't just a quick-fix bandage. Some of you have made some serious lifestyle changes. And while they might not always have been easy, I challenge you to say that they weren't worth it. Because those changes were for you, and YOU ARE WORTH IT!

That's the main thing that I want you to remind yourself whenever you start to stray from this path of health and wellness; that you are doing this for yourself and that you are worth it! Do not let anyone tell you otherwise. Don't let that little voice inside your head tell you otherwise, either. You know, the one who makes you feel guilty for putting yourself first. You are no good to anyone else if you aren't good to yourself first! Remember this!

If you do stray, don't beat yourself up over it. You've just strayed, you're not lost. The path is still in sight; you just need to get back on it.

Like the shampoo bottle says: "lather, rinse, repeat." Re-read this. It's not *War and Peace*, so it isn't going to take long to repeat. Keep the information always fresh in your mind.

Pay it forward. Share the information that you have learned with those you love who might need it. Give them a copy of this program. Take them for a walk with you. Tell YOUR story to help others not feel alone in their journey to health. Sharing is caring!

And please share with me! I LOVE hearing your success stories! Contact me at lara@yolarates.com

Be happy!

Lara

Lara Foldvari is just like you. Really. She has been there.

Like you, she is not a bikini model or an Olympic lifter. But she has struggled with her weight and her health, so she knows what you are going through.

Lara has been published in a handful of tattoo enthusiast magazines and is the author of *Just a Good Cook...* She is certified by AFAA and ACE as a Group Fitness Instructor and Personal Trainer, by NESTA as a Lifestyle and Weight Management Specialist, and NASM as a Fitness Nutrition Specialist. She teaches YoLarates™ and Zumba® classes at private studios and community centers in the Cheshire, CT area.

Lara lives in Cheshire with her Man, their Storkie (a Yorkie with 8-inch legs!), and a flock of hens.

You can contact Lara at lara@yolarates.com. Check out her website at www.yolarates.com.